The Smoothie Diet 21-Day Rapid Weight L

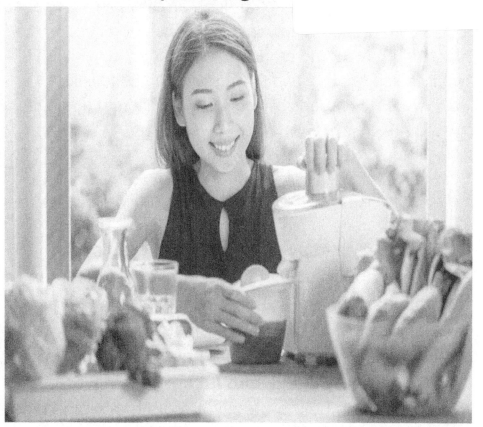

Presented by: Baiad Mengud

www.baiadsmoothiediet.com

Copyright © 2022

Introduction.

When it comes to an easy and rapid way to lose weight and burn fat without hunger, drinking Green Smoothies is one of the best ways to achieve your weight loss goals. Green Smoothies are so easy to make. It also tastes great and not only does it help you to lose weight and burn fat but drinking Green Smoothies can help protect you from many diseases.

Table of Contents

About The Author.

I am Baiad Mengud, living in Kuching City, Malaysia. I had been working with a private company for more than 20 years already. I like hot and spicy food.

I am passionate about health and fitness especially on losing weight. I found out that losing weight with a smoothie Diet is a fantastic way as it is easy to prepare anywhere you like.

The Smoothie Diet 21-Day Program For Rapid Weight Loss

The 21 Day Smoothie Diet Rapid Weight Loss Program is among the most famous smoothie diets. It provides a wide range of health advantages, significantly affecting both health and wellbeing and resulting in major changes in fitness and health.With Smoothie Diet you will be able to achieve your goal easily even if you are living a very busy lifestyle.

Nowadays there are many ways and programs to lose weight and people spend thousands of dollars by going to the gym and hiring personal trainers, hoping to lose weight. However if you are looking for a weight loss program based on green smoothies, I recommend you to check out smoothie expert [Drew's 21-Day Smoothie Diet Programs](). It's the form of an ebook program.

Before you start, you have to do a three-day detox. It involves the use of the "3-day Smoothie Detox Program", a bonus you get after purchasing. The detox prepares your body for the actual 21-day program.

Why a Smoothie Diet?

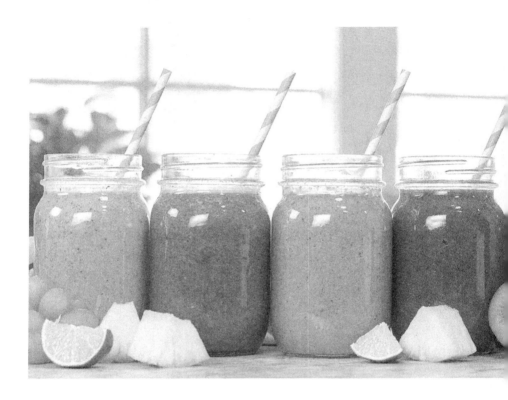

Green smoothies are nutrients rich and loaded with vitamins. It is easy to prepare in the morning or even a few minutes before you start to drink. The basic concept of the smoothie diet is like a meal replacement. You replace unhealthy fat gaining food with healthy smoothies.

The best part of The Smoothie Diet is that you can use it for as long as you need, to lose as much weight as you want. The 21-Day program makes it super simple to continue using everything you learn in the first 3 weeks to extend the program for the next few weeks or even months. And each additional week will be just as enjoyable as the first three! The goal is to give you all the tools you need to continue losing weight and getting healthy for as long as you need to.

Unlike other diets, the 21 days program is only the beginning to a lifetime of better health and a slimmer body. After a few weeks, the cravings for sweets and junk foods will essentially disappear. This makes it very easy to keep the weight off. In fact, most people love smoothies so much and they don't want to give up after 21 days. Some clients said this is a complete life-transformation program.

If you don't have a lot of time in the day, then this program is still PERFECT to follow because the program is super simple and takes minutes a day. The recipes are quick to make and you can either enjoy it right away or take them with you.

What do you get from the 21 Day Smoothie Diet Program?

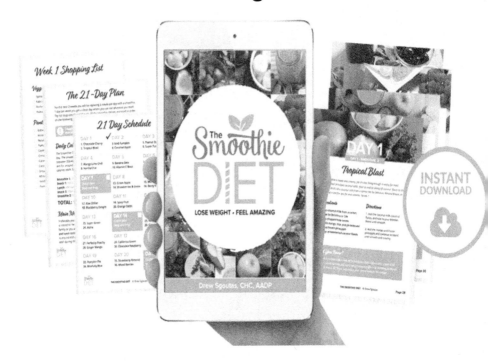

This 21 Days Smoothie Diet program will give you detailed meal plans along with delicious smoothie recipes, grocery shopping list and healthy eating guide.

Plus, you get kids friendly smoothie recipes as well. You will also get insider tips on making smoothies and spend less time in the kitchen. Besides, you also get diabetes friendly + gluten free smoothie recipes to follow the program.

Benefits of 21 Days Smoothie Diet Program.

A 21 day weight loss plan that tells you which smoothie to have when for maximum results

GUIDE 3-DAY Smoothie DIET Detox

Lose Weight & feel Amazing

just for you

GET $10 OFF
LIMITED-TIME OFFER! – ONLY $47 $37
60 DAY

Smoothie diet is not as difficult as you think. It's only a liquid diet from green vegetables and fruits. Adding smoothies into some of your meals would help you to lose weight quickly and easily.

Below are the benefits you get.

- You can easily follow a diet plan along with 36 smoothie recipes to help you to lose weight.
- You get personal access to health coach Drew for any questions during the program.
- Low price compared to any diet programs.
- No-risk, money back guarantee if you do not find it useful.

Other potential benefits of drinking smoothies.

- Increases consumption of fruits and vegetables.
- Increases fiber intake.
- Can be a meal replacement.
- Can provide a nutritional balance of fats, protein, carbohydrates, vitamins, and minerals.
- Helps manage food cravings.
- You will get 2 bonuses after purchasing.

Bonus # 1.

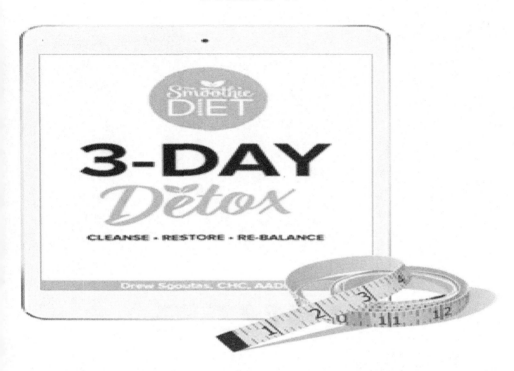

This Detox program is easily worth the price of the whole program. This is something you can do before you start the 21-Day program to help clear out the "cobwebs" and get your body ready for optimal results. It can also be used anytime you want to lose a quick few pounds. The great thing is that you will see almost instant weight loss results. One of the clients lost 3 Lbs in 3 Days with this detox program. The program includes 3 days of 3 specially designed meal replacement detox smoothie recipes, a complete shopping list for everything you need, as well as your choice of 2 recipe options.

Bonus # 2.

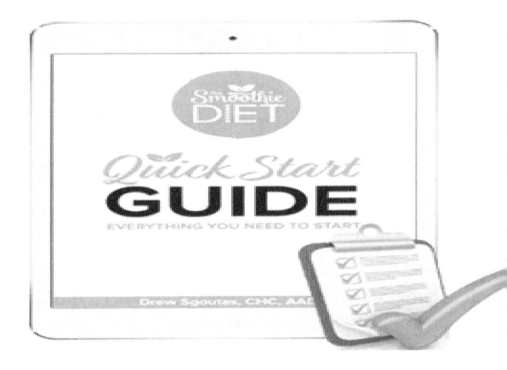

If you're anything like me, you wanna get right to the good stuff! I designed this guide to be an easy reference you can print out and start using right away without needing to read the longer core guide. It's a condensed version of the core guide that contains the 3-week schedule, shopping lists, prep guide, and smoothie recipes. This is a fast track "to do" list that will help you start enjoying the benefits of the program from the very first instant you download it.

Health Benefits Of Smoothie Diet.

1. Helpful In Rapid Weight Loss.

The Smoothie Diet can help you lose a lot of weight because a green smoothie normally comprises a lot of green vegetables and fruits. Its efficiency is boosted by the absence of fat-adding foods like dairy which contribute unnecessary fats and calories to your body. By consuming the smoothies diet it reduces the intake of extra calories.

2.Boost The Digestive System And Gut Health.

The high amount of fiber in the smoothies diet is very useful for boosting and improving your digestion system. It helps in regular bowel movements.

3.Boosts/Improves Immunity.

When followed properly, The smoothies diet plan will result in a better immune system. According to studies, green smoothies with a lot of green vegetables, include the nutrients that your immune system needs. Vitamin C from vegetables and fruits,helps to maintain the immune system. It also helps in the fighting against infections.

4. Low Cholesterol.

From your smoothie diet, useful chemicals help prevent the formation of fatty deposits on artery walls, lowering the risk of heart disease.

5.Low Chances Of Cardiac Diseases.

When it comes to health and wellness, the smoothie diet is one of the healthiest and safest options. It includes leafy greens which are considered to be high in antioxidants including Vitamin C and beta-carotene. These antioxidants are well-known for their ability to prevent and reverse oxidative damage produced by free radicals. As a result of low cholesterol in your body, the chances of cardiac diseases decrease automatically.

6. Good For Mental Health.

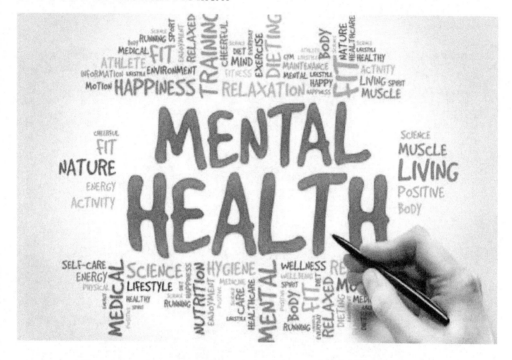

If you are uncomfortable with your weight, you may feel compelled and you will try to avoid public appearances because you are self-conscious. However, if you begin to lose weight, you will feel more confident in yourself.

7.Anti - Aging

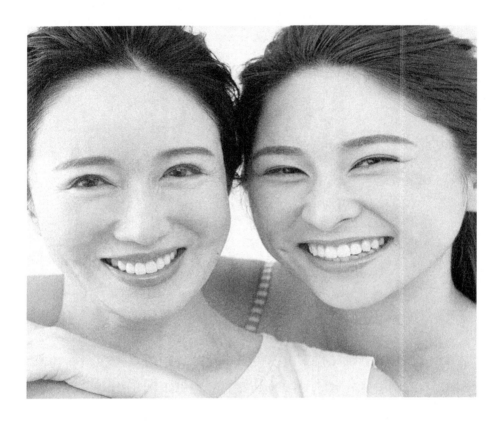

Green smoothies are a great source of these anti-aging enzymes.

You don't only get clearer skin, but the nutrients in green smoothies also help to boost production of collagen, creating firmer and younger looking skin.

Apples, strawberries and oranges are great choices to add to your smoothie.

Tips To make basic smoothies.

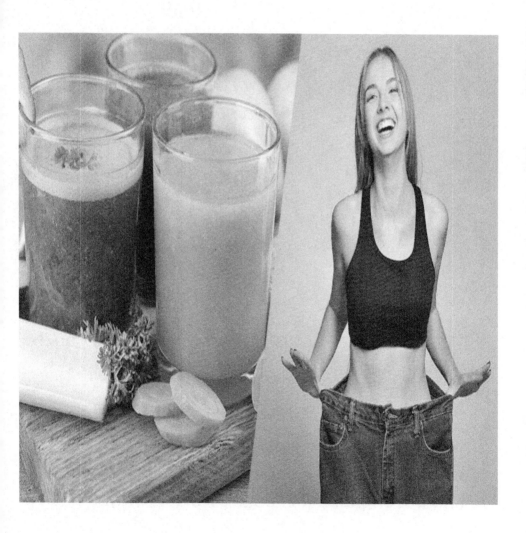

Below are a few of my favorite tips to share with you how to make the best creamy and healthy smoothies:

1.Use frozen fruit.

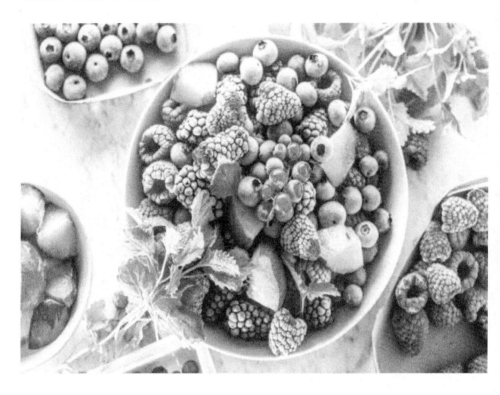

Using frozen fruit is best because it helps to keep the smoothie cold and thick.

2.Add more liquid.

To add more liquid when your smoothie is too thick or not fully blended. High powered blenders tend to blend frozen fruit much better. However if you have a regular or personal size blender, you need to add more milk.

3.Blend low then blend high.

Start the blender on low speed, then gradually increase to high speed to help to blend all the ingredients. Then turn the blender power to low speed.

4.Sweeten to your desired taste.

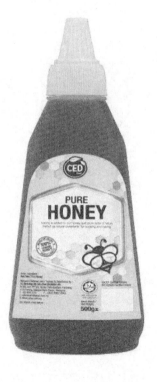

If a smoothie doesn't taste sweet enough, you can add a 1/2 tablespoon of honey, pure maple syrup or 1 pitted Medjool date.

5.Choose your own milk flavor.

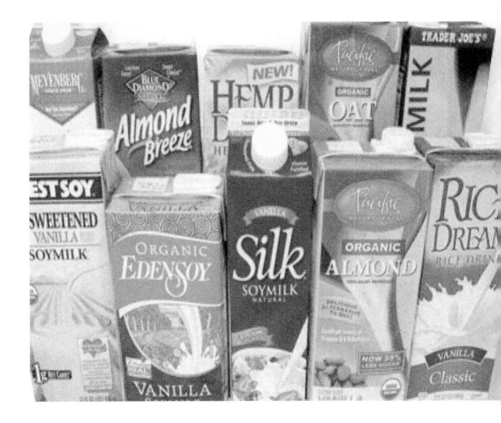

Feel free to use any milk based on your own taste and preferences. Almond milk tends to have a neutral taste in smoothies. Coconut milk will add a more tropical and creamy flavor and regular milk will add a boost of protein.

Testimonials.

Below are a few testimonials from health expert Drew's clients that he has published. Results show that the program is real and it works!

Danielle Lost 8 Pounds in 1 Week!

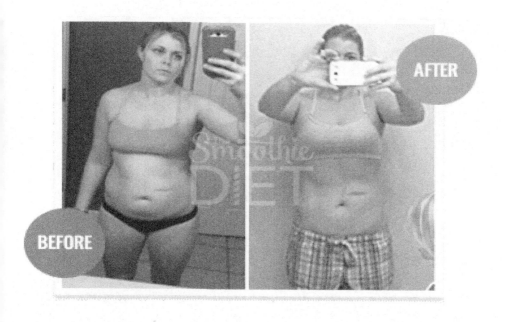

"Getting into this diet was so easy and the results were so fast. After only 1 week on the Smoothie Diet I weighed myself

and realized I had lost 8 pounds! I feel better and more confident than I have in a very long time, I don't have to suck in my stomach to button my pants anymore and I still have to stop doing a double take everytime I walk in front of a mirror."

Danielle Lost 8 Pounds in 1 Week!

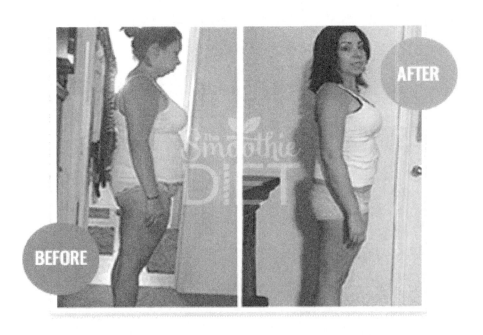

"Getting into this diet was so easy and the results were so fast. After only 1 week on the Smoothie Diet I weighed myself and realized I had lost 8 pounds! I feel better and more confident than I have in a very long time, I don't have to suck in my stomach to button my pants anymore and I still have to stop doing a double take everytime I walk in front of a mirror"

Jade lost 12 Pounds in 21 Days!

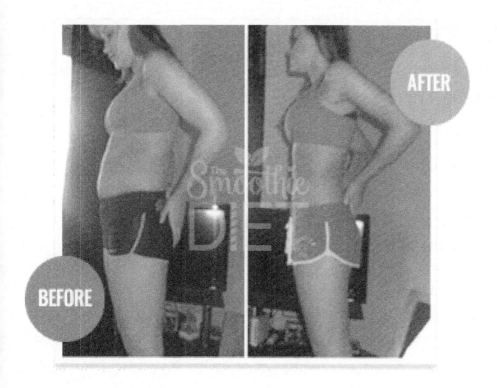

"I've been trying forever to lose the last 10-15 lbs. and tone up and that's exactly what happened so I am very happy. I feel great about myself, I don't find myself holding in my belly anymore and feel confident about myself and people have noticed that about me too...and my love handles are gone! I couldn't be happier with this whole program and I definitely recommend this to anyone looking to lose a little or lose a lot."

Conclusion.

The 21-Day Smoothie Diet Program is a good diet program for weight loss. It has more benefits in losing weight than harm.

And somehow if the smoothie diet 21 days rapid weight loss programme doesn't work for you, you will get a risk-free 2-month return and refund assurance. It's a win-win situation.

This smoothie diet program has everything laid out step-by-step for you to start losing weight today and tomorrow.Whether you are just trying to lose the last 5-10 lbs or you want to lose 30 lbs or more,I invite you to try the Smoothie Diet 21-Day Program For Rapid Weight Loss to see how effective detox smoothies for weight loss can be.

Printed in Great Britain
by Amazon

21714987R00020